grown-up
&
gorgeous

in your 40s

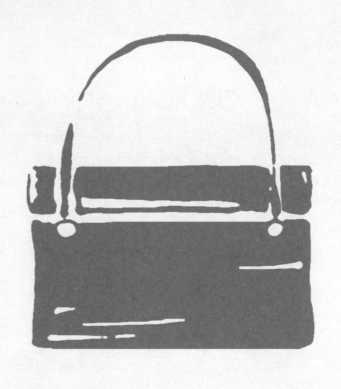

grown-up & gorgeous

in your 40s

Pamela Robson

EBURY
PRESS

Acknowledgements: Dr Mary Dingley, President of the Australasian Society of Cosmetic Physicians; Tanja Mrnjaus, ID Couture, Melbourne, Sydney and Brisbane; Dr Shane Rea, Barshop Institute for Longevity and Aging Studies, University of Texas; Ken Gordon & Toni Adams, Musculo-Skeletal Clinic, Spring Hill, Queensland; Dr Cathy Gaulton, Pacific Cosmetic Surgery, Brisbane, Queensland; Jean Hailes Foundation; Wellesley College Biology Department, Maryland; American Academy of Peridontology

Contents

You're not quite sure how it happened, but suddenly you're forty. You've just reached a stage in life when you're confidently managing it all, then the first signs of ageing start to appear. You're beginning to feel just slightly less than gorgeous. The trouble is that age creeps up on you. While you are concentrating on work, kids, and all the issues thrown up by the roller-coaster ride we call life, everything is quietly but resolutely travelling downwards. These days you can probably finally afford to spend a bit of money on yourself but finding the time to do it is the hard part. And this is the decade when getting healthy, active, live-minded and, above all, looking good is going to pay the biggest dividends for the future. Don't fret. You're not alone. In the terrific, terrifying 21st century, you can be anything you want to be . . . and here's how.

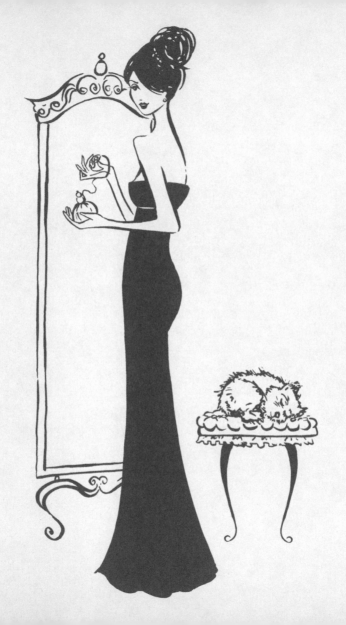

Beauty

Your 40s is the most time-poor of all the decades. For a generation that's made an art-form out of multi-tasking there's little space left in the day to indulge in a facial or pedicure. But this is also the stage of life when a few well-chosen treatments and products can make all the difference as to how you look in the coming years.

Beauty can be time-consuming, but only if you let it. Sure, there are women for whom make-up is pure therapy, and who look forward to their skincare regimen almost as a form of meditation, but for most of us beauty survival is about prioritising. This means finding products and treatment that are evidence-based and can make a real difference. It's also about seeking professional help. In the long run, this can save you time, money, and very likely your sanity.

Your new best friends

A hairdresser who has that rare trio of qualities: experience,
skill and the ability to be tactfully frank with you

IIIII

The guru at your nearest eyebrow bar

IIIII

A fashion stylist or image consultant who can makeover
your wardrobe, take you shopping for the right clothes,
and ultimately take the strain off your wallet

IIIII

An exercise physiologist – they're tertiary-trained in how
the body works

IIIII

A musculo-skeletal therapist who understands 'computer back'

IIIII

A dietician who talks common sense

IIIII

A skilled and experienced cosmetic physician

IIIII

A properly trained cosmetic plastic surgeon who is
experienced in the procedures that you're seeking

IIIII

Make-up – less is more

The older we get the more we need to edit our make-up. Tempting though it is, far from disguising imperfections, thicker foundations and lots of eye make-up can actually make you look older. Twenty-year-olds with radiant complexions can look stunning as painted dolls in the pages of the glossies. Forty-year-olds definitely do not – especially in broad daylight. There are some great new foundations and tinted moisturisers aimed at creating a flawless, natural, complexion. You might also need hydrating make-up.

Back to the Stone Age

The 'big new thing' is mineral make-up. It's actually been around for 30 years but has just been rediscovered because it's light, translucent, and good for ageing skins, with mineral particles that deflect the light. Part of its appeal is that it's seen as being more natural than conventional make-up, with fewer chemicals. Many brands contain zinc oxide which also offers natural UVA-UVB protection.

Be primed

Use a primer under your foundation. As the name suggests, primers act just like paint primers, preparing the skin surface and filling in lines. Containing silicon, they make the skin feel soft but not sticky; foundation glides on and lasts longer.

TRY THIS:

- *Apply a creamy concealer that's about two shades lighter than your skin tone to any dark circles under your eyes. This instantly makes you look fresher and more youthful.*

- *Identify the enemy. The sun can age you faster than just about anything on the planet. Sun damage accounts for an estimated 90 per cent of the lines, wrinkles, folds and crepeyness we develop. Make this your mantra: I will use sunblock, and wear a hat and sunglasses.*

- *Use a good foundation that contains an SPF and follow doctors' advice that you use a separate sunscreen underneath. The ones made for babies are a good choice – they're light and non-allergenic. Put it on 20 minutes before your foundation.*

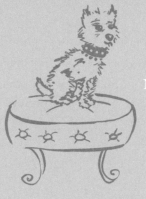

Now is the time to jettison the thick eyeliner and heavy shadow. Drooping and crepey upper eyelids do not fare well under layers of paint. Even if you've always been a Cleopatra at heart, you'll look younger and fresher with minimal eye make-up. Heavy eye make-up can give a hard look. Let's be honest here: it's the stuff of drag queens.

Soften the shadows

Keep eyeliner as close to the lashes as your dexterity will allow. Go for natural colours of shadow – a smudge of something smoky is about as far as you should go; forget the three colours on the lid with a pearly white on the brow bone – it's too fussy and very 80s. Don't be tempted to buy cheap products – powders that can dry and cake and creams that can clog in the lines. Buy good brands and translucent powders that give your lids a dewy look.

Underneath the arches

These unsung heroes of facial balance are finally being recognised for the important role they play. A pair of well-tinted, classically shaped brows with just the right degree of arch and length can frame the face and bring out the colour and depth of the eyes. Brow stylists and brow bars are springing up all over the place as we realise that expert help is critical in establishing the right shape and line.

TRY THIS:

If you have sensitive skin, before you pluck your brows use an antiseptic skin solution made for cuts and abrasions that contains Lignocaine for pain relief.

As we age and our facial hair greys, our features become less distinct. It's value for money to have a regular professional lash and brow tint and eyebrow reshape.

If you have naturally sparse brows, try brushing in some fine powdered shadow – it's easier than drawing a line and can look more natural.

The debate around plucking versus waxing has pros and cons on both sides, so leave it up to your stylist.

Eyebrow tattooing has come a long way. If your eyebrows have dropped or become too thin, consider having natural-looking colour implants by a recommended cosmetic tattooist.

Bonzer bronzer

A bit of a tan can take years off the way you look,
but less is more when it comes to bronzer. The trick
is to pick the right colour and brush it on quickly and
lightly with a deft hand. Too dark a shade and bronzer
clings to the fine lines and wrinkles like contours on
a map; too red and you'll look like Geronimo. The
foolproof way is to go for a neutral undertone, flicking
it swiftly under the cheekbone and up towards the
temples. With what's left on the brush, sweep along
the jawline and across the forehead. Try a few shades
before you buy and choose the one that looks
most natural. Better still,
play it safe with a
matte bronzer
that creates a
more subtle
glow.

Blush a little

Unless you are a professional make-up artist, forget trying to sculpt your face with blusher. Choose a colour that's not too dark for your skin tone – peach suits most people – and make sure it's a cream blusher rather than powder. Dot it onto the apple – the fattest part – of your cheek and use a little dampened sponge to blend it back towards your hairline. The idea is a delicate youthful glow – not pink or orange streaks.

Light years ahead

One of the best new technologies to come out of the cosmetics lab in recent years is the illuminator. Wear it under your foundation to give a youthful glow and to help minimise lines, blotches and other imperfections. Illuminators contain mica particles that deflect light away from the skin. Once you start using an illuminator you won't know how you got along without it.

Lip reading

Abandon dark lipsticks in favour of lighter colours that won't travel by osmosis up those vertical lines we call smokers' lines. Darker colours make your lips look thinner. It's the same reason we wear black pants.

Be choosy about which of the long-lasting lippies to wear. Early ones were incredibly drying and shrivelled lips at the very touch. There's a whole new generation of longer-lasters out there that are creamier and come with a separate lip gloss.

The older you are the creamier your lipstick needs to be.

★

During the day try using just a gloss on its own for a natural look.

★

Match your lip liner as closely as possible to your lipstick. Never use a dark lip liner: when your lipstick wears off it looks just plain silly.

Flash 'em

One of the simplest things you can do to take 10 years off your appearance is have your teeth whitened. It looks healthy and sexy, and it can boost your self-confidence because your mouth and teeth are the first things that anyone looks at when they meet you. Your dentist can make custom-fitted trays that you fill with a bleaching gel and wear at home, or teeth whitening can be done in the dental surgery with bleach applied under a laser or light (a more expensive but quicker option).

The skin you're in

There is a saying in cosmetic medical circles: 'the quickest way to age is to lie in the sun and smoke', because the enemies of the skin are UV rays and the chemicals in cigarettes. The skin rebuilds itself on a continual basis and maintaining it is all about the way we live.

Here are the five most important things you must do to ensure your skin stays looking fresh in your 40s:

1 **PROTECT** your skin from the sun. This is THE most important thing. And it's not just about your face; a 30-year-old face above 80-year-old cleavage is not a good look, and the skin on your chest is much harder to rejuvenate.

2 **QUIT** smoking. If you haven't found a reason to give up yet – other than dying – just remember that smoking affects your skin at the cell level and can make you look very old before your time.

3 **EAT WELL:** A diet rich in fruit, vegetables, whole grains and lean protein will help you get the vitamin C (for collagen production), antioxidants (for anti-ageing) and essential fatty acids your skin needs to be at its best. Hydration is essential for great skin, so drink plenty of fluids.

4 **EXFOLIATE:** This is a fundamental of skin care for both face and body. Polishing off the outermost skin cells stimulates the cell renewal process and helps achieve a healthy glow, while also revving up collagen production. Use a facial exfoliant (a cream with dry-skin-removing ingredients) every three days, and use a cream exfoliant, body brush, loofah or mitt in the shower every day.

5 **TAKE ACTION** if you feel like you're losing the battle! For repair and maintenance, there are plenty of new technologically driven treatments that can help you avoid a trip to the operating theatre, or at least stave it off for a few more years. For the best and latest in low-invasive treatments, read on . . .

The truth about face creams

Whether you spend $40 or $400 on a pot of face cream, you need to know that they are limited in what they can do. Realistically, what most do is to hold the moisture in. They cannot put moisture back into the skin. Here's why: the outer layer of the skin is the body's main barrier against infection. It's designed to stop bacteria and other nasties getting through. It's also waterproof, while allowing the body to sweat and lose heat when it needs to cool down. What this all means is that the molecules in a face cream have to be oh-so-tiny if they are to penetrate the skin barrier. Very few creams have ingredients that can accomplish this.

Having said that, as we get older we all must use a cream to keep the moisture in because our complexions become dryer. By our 40s our bodies are less efficient at producing collagen, elastin and hyaluronic acid – the skin's building blocks. The middle layer of skin becomes less dense, collapses and forms wrinkles and the cells in the outer layer become brittle and less able to hold moisture.

as we get older our complexions become dryer

The body makes collagen from vitamin C. One scientist with too much time on his hands has worked out that it takes about 60 milligrams of vitamin C to make 2 grams of collagen. All creams that promise to put vitamin C or collagen or elastin back into your skin cannot do what they claim. Ask a dermatologist or cosmetic doctor for advice.

21st-century beauty arsenal

Remember when a skincare regimen meant a packet of cotton wool balls and three bottles with labels that said cleanser, toner and moisturiser? Well, now it's more likely to be about chemicals, lasers and radio frequency, and your 40s is about the time to get started.

The whole push in cosmetic surgery these days is to avoid it – surgery that is. Some of the best and brightest alternatives are:

★ Tretinoin (Retin A and Retrieve) peels the outer layer of the skin, encouraging faster cell turnover, and activates a genetic 'switch' that stimulates production of collagen and elastin. You should use it sparingly and gradually; and because it peels the skin, you must avoid the sun.

★ Exfoliants and vitamin creams for skin maintenance.

★ Hyaluronic acid pinprick injections to aid hydration.

★ Botox. Long used in the upper part of the face to freeze frown lines and crows' feet, now doctors also inject this chemical into muscles of the brow to create a very effective brow lift. Used on either side of the mouth it relieves that depressed, down-in-the-mouth look. Necks are also being targeted, to relax visible tense muscles and improve posture.

★ New generation skin resurfacers to improve/maintain skin quality.

★ Temporary and permanent fillers for lines and lips.

★ Cosmetic fillers to sculpt faces and add lost volume.

★ Radiofrequency treatment to tighten up loose skin.

BE CAREFUL: With Botox, you get what you pay for: a cheap deal won't necessarily deliver the best results. The practitioner might be using less Botox, or they may not have much experience yet.

Skin smoothers

There is a battalion of new technology out there to help improve skin quality, each with its own area of specialty. The latest technologies try to match the skin rejuvenation properties of earlier CO_2 and erbium lasers that were very effective and most popular a decade ago, but without the complications that these first machines produced – especially hypopigmentation, a permanent whitening of the skin. Some new technologies aim to do this by reaching the lower levels of the skin while leaving the surface intact; others try to achieve comparable results through a series of less invasive treatments instead of a one-off procedure. They include:

Plasma resurfacing is the very latest skin treatment technology, involving a stream of nitrogen converted into a plasma of ionised gas, which is fired at the skin to remove the surface. The plasma does, however, induce heat in the skin and some patients find this difficult. It's usually a one-off procedure.

IPL (Intense Pulsed Light) is a broad-spectrum light that's perfect if you just want a light polish and to get rid of blotchiness. Good for removing freckles, brown age spots and broken capillaries. IPL is offered by medical practices and beauty salons and is dubbed a 'lunchtime' treatment – which means you can go straight back to your normal daily routine afterwards.

Fraxel laser treats the skin pixel fashion, triggering the body's natural healing process and speeding up the production of collagen and new, healthy skin cells. This is the latest laser technology and the first that has shown promise for treating stretch marks. It's good on old acne scars and can be used on the neck, chest and arms. Effects continue for three to six months after the treatment, so you won't see the best results straightaway.

Radiofrequency treatment (Thermage) is the only non-surgical procedure for tightening loose skin. It uses mono-polar radiofrequency to pump heat into the sub dermal layers of the skin while cooling the outer layer. It's good for lifting sagging jowls and jawlines, upper eyes and brows and it is effective on cellulite.

As we age, some things perversely
start to shrink. We lose bone – including
the skull – we lose muscle volume, and we lose
fat from our face. We also produce less collagen
and elastin, the skin's building blocks. What this all
means is that the middle layer of the skin becomes less
dense and wrinkles form. The cheek fat pads descend, which
means we get folds and a less-defined jawline. And our lips
get thinner and those vertical smokers' lines start to appear.

Up the volume

So, one of our main aims is to increase volume in the
face. Cosmetic fillers for lips and lines can be temporary
(hyaluronic acid products) or more permanent (gels like
Aquamid). Practitioners often have allegiance to one
company and will sometimes echo the qualities of
their brand over the others, so shop around
and do lots of research.

Hyaluronic fillers are now also being used to add volume to the face through injection deep under the skin, to help define a jawline, relieve hollows beneath the eyes, or build up cheekbones. The effects can last for a year or two. Used together with a Botox brow lift, such fillers can alleviate the need for a surgical brow lift. Sculptra, a synthetic polylactic acid, stimulates the body to produce its own collagen, so for facial sculpting it can be injected into any area that needs volume.

Drooping eyelids can be remedied surgically by removing a small amount of skin in the crease of the lid. Swelling and bruising are common afterwards, but this is regarded as a straightforward procedure and results are generally very good. Undereye bags can be corrected in another straightforward procedure.

For adjustments below the neck, diet and exercise can be backed up with liposuction or lipolysis. But let's get one thing straight: liposuction is not a weight

Body work

loss treatment, it reshapes your body. When your body gets back to normal a few months after your procedure you'll find that you weigh much the same as you did before – but you will be a different shape. It is not uncommon for women to remark that following liposuction of the lower body – hips, abdomen etc – they find that they carry more weight up top; as the weight redistributes itself, you may go up a size or two in bra cups. It's great for reducing big thighs, tummies, waists, love handles and squishy under-bra-strap backs.

Liposuction is very skill-dependent, with results varying according to the skill and artistry of the surgeon and the quality of the patient's skin.

Lipolysis (where a chemical is injected to dissolve fat deposits) is an alternative to liposuction, especially where there are small areas of fat to remove. It offers a greater degree of control – which makes it particularly suitable for the face and neck.

A little lift

By the time you've reached your mid 40s you've probably found yourself – more than once – in front of a mirror pulling up those sagging cheeks and jowls and speculating on how you would look with the help of a little surgery. We've mostly all been there. Finding the right facelift isn't easy. There are as many types of facelift as there are surgeons performing them: from low-invasive mini-lift and S lifts (which, many surgeons will tell you, are not long-lasting), to mid facelifts and deep SMAS facelifts where the surgeon lifts the underlying tissue and drapes the skin back over it. The results depend on the techniques used, the style preferred by the surgeon, and the quality of the original material – your face. But be warned: even the best facelifts drop over time, so be prepared to have it redone after about 10 years.

Cosmetic surgery is unregulated in Australia, so it can't be stressed enough that you need to do your homework when deciding on a procedure – surgical or otherwise. Just because you like the style of the surgeon, it doesn't mean they're brilliant with a scalpel. Don't rush into it and do plenty of research.

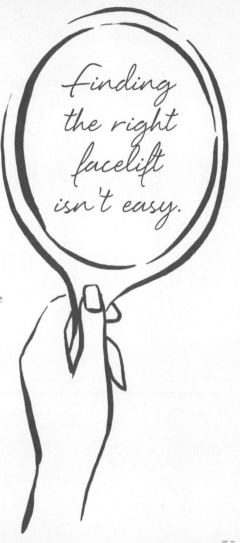

finding the right facelift isn't easy.

Hair today . . .

Often in the rush to rejuvenate
our faces we forget that our
hair also ages and needs a little
help. Just like the skin, the scalp
starts to dry and the hair strands
become less supple. If you've been
a keen sun-bather, had your hair
regularly coloured, straightened,
permed or blow-dried, your hair
will probably be physically older
than its chronological age. One of
the best things you can do for your
hair is to wear a hat in the sun.

...*gone tomorrow*

If you've found that your hair is getting thinner, you're not alone. By 35, an estimated 40 per cent of men and women will have started to experience hair loss. While there is a huge industry devoted to male hair loss, not much is known about women's thinning problems. The pattern of baldness is different between the sexes and there is evidence that various enzymes, hormone receptors and blockers may be at work in women. Auto-immune and hormone disorders cause hair loss. Sometimes women can lose hair temporarily after illness, surgery or pregnancy, or following a stressful event such as divorce. Nutrition also plays a big part, and iron deficiency and even crash dieting can cause hair loss.

The best place to start is your GP and dermatologist.

Faking volume

To a large extent, beauty is all about looking healthy, and healthy hair is about volume. You can fake thicker hair through conditioning, cut and style. Your hairdresser will be able to advise you on conditioning treatments and there are a number that you can try at home. There are also quite a few new 'anti-ageing' shampoos on the market that promise to address ageing hair shafts and drying scalps.

You can fake thicker hair through conditioning, cut and style.

Style

Healthy shiny
hair is youthful;
hair that is
plastered down
and heavy with
product isn't.
Choose a style
that has bounce
and moves. Have the
hair around your face
layered to give it a lift. Go
for softer styles with fewer
sharp angles. Consider
a soft but fine fringe
– it can hide a
multitude of sins. If you wear your hair
long, make sure it's got volume and
bounce. Long thin hair is not a good look
at any age.

The rules about hair colour

Go two shades lighter and warmer. Softer, lighter colours are kinder to the ageing face. Ashes bring out the grey. Avoid blocks of dark colour that can throw dark shadows into lines and wrinkles. Instead opt for foils and streaks. Sometimes hair that is greying also turns coarser and wiry. Colouring products can help address this.

Hair generally begins to lose its colour between the ages of 34 and 42. There is no difference between dark and fair hair and it's generally thought to be mainly down to our genes, but environment, lifestyle – especially stress – and nutrition play a part. Recently, skin cancer research scientists stumbled on how and why it happens. It's all due to the gradual dying off of adult stem cells called melanocytes that provide the hair follicles with pigment. They become less efficient and make mistakes as they age and as a result the hair also loses its shiny, healthy and youthful appearance. Scientists elsewhere are working on ways to regenerate the melanocytes in hair. There are products that are already being used to reinvigorate melanocytes to treat skin hypopigmentation (loss of colour).

No more grey?

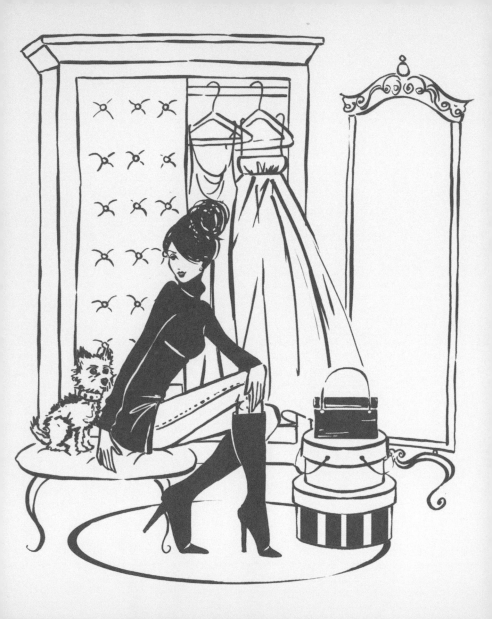

Wardrobe

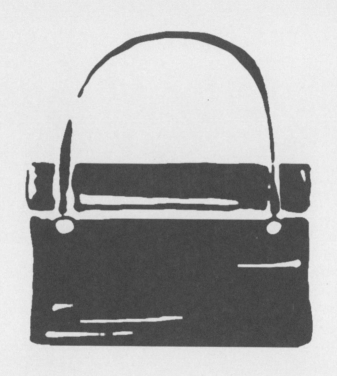

44

By 40 you probably have a good idea of the shapes and hues that look right for your figure and colouring. But you probably don't have the time to research the new season's styles or shop. If you're like most people, the chances are that you've gained a few kilos – and generally in the wrong places. This probably means your fashion goals have shifted along with your waistline, which can leave you prone to playing it super-safe and coming across style-wise as just a tad boring. Erring on the side of caution makes it easy to get stuck in a fashion time warp. But here's the best thing about reaching your 40s: by now it's probably struck home that just because it's in every shop it doesn't mean you have to wear it. Each season, pick and choose what you like and what suits you, and don't be afraid to let a so-called 'must-have' shape go by. Instead, spend up on accessories to keep your look current until something that appeals *and* flatters comes along.

Most of us put on a few kilos in our 40s, especially around the middle – which means we start combing the shops for items that give us a longer, leaner look. The trick is to stay current while finding clothes that flatter the less good bits and play up the quite good bits. The areas you want to downplay should be dressed simply, steering away from lots of detail that draws the eye. As we all know, dark colours make us look slimmer, which is why a few pairs of black pants and dark jeans are the staple of any 40-something's wardrobe.

It's the *silhouette*, silly

Each season fashion designers come up with the new silhouette – the outline of how clothes will look on the catwalk and in the high street. It could be a short jacket with wide pants or a long top with tight jeans. It's a good idea to start thinking in terms of outline shapes and identifying those garments that create the best outline shape for your body. Are you small topped/

wide hipped; wide shouldered/ narrow hipped; large breasted/ narrow hipped; hour-glass; petite; or voluptuous? Once you've established what shape you are, research the garments and the combinations that flatter you most. Think about the shape of the pants that best suit you – narrow, wide, flat-fronted, side-zipped, three-quarter? Think about where the jacket hem should reach – never your widest part. Shop for items that enhance your good bits: neck and shoulders, cleavage or legs. Choose fabrics that drape and skim where they should.

And most of all don't worry. Whatever your shape, whatever your size, there is a garment out there that can make you look fabulous.

TRY THIS:
If you are putting on weight around your middle, minimise it and achieve a smooth line with flat-fronted skirts and pants that sit just below your natural waist. Side-zipped pants and jeans are fab for flattering even the most difficult stomachs and bottoms.

This is something all the experts agree on: the perfect skirt should end just at the top of the knee, or, if you want to be a little more conservative, the middle of the knee. If your skirt hits mid-calf, visually it cuts your legs in half and makes them look wider than they are. Unless you want to look like you are trying too hard, don't wear super-short skirts.

The perfect skirt length

The A-line skirt – one that flares out slightly from the waistline to the hem – is generally regarded as being flattering for most figures, but particularly for those of us with small tops and big hips. A straight skirt is another stylish option as long as it isn't too tight – a good rule to follow for all clothing decisions. If you are slim and want to emphasise whatever curves you do have, go for the pencil skirt, or a straight skirt that flares out at the hem.

A straight skirt is another stylish option

Getting it together

There is a very simple rule for pairing tops and skirts, and again, it's all about proportion and balance. If you wear a loose-fitting top, go for a neat-fitting skirt. If you are wearing a floaty or otherwise voluminous skirt, stick to a tight-fitting top. If both pieces are big and loose you'll look like you're wearing a sack. If both are too tight, you'll look like a tart.

It's a common fashion mistake: wearing oversized T-shirts and tops in the belief that they disguise lumps and bumps. Sadly, they only make you look huge. A smaller and

Tops that trim

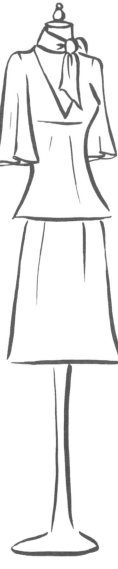

slightly more fitted top (not skin-tight) will skim over curves and flatter your shape – not put a bag over it. You need a shape that slims and elongates your figure. A tunic that ends just below the bottom is generally flattering, as is a top cut to the high hip bone – which can be flattering over skirts.

Tunic tops, tops in draping fabrics, or crossover tops are all workable options. When it comes to T-shirts, just because they're a basic don't go for the cheapest and make sure you try a few on. Some have wider armhole sizes, others fit better across the chest, and some have a longer neck-to-hem length. They're all different.

If you have large breasts, be careful the top doesn't pull at the back and accentuate any under-bra strap squishyness. Layering is an excellent option: for example, find a lightweight bolero or jacket to disguise a chubby back. Unless you have great arms, it's safer to stick to tops with some sort of sleeve.

Necklines that flatter

If you have big breasts, a V-neck is more flattering than a round neck, which will make you look even more top heavy. The V-shape also helps to elongate a short neck. If you have small breasts go for round necks and boat necks that draw the eye upwards. But avoid boat necks if you have wide shoulders or a thick neck. Instead, a round or 'jewel' (slightly wider) neckline can be really flattering.

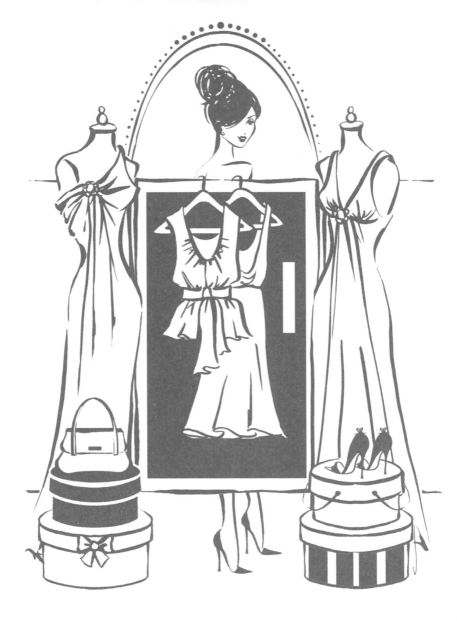

Colour coded

Nothing says more about your personality than the colours you wear. By your 40s you'll have a fair idea of what works best for you. There'll be those that cause people to say: Wow, you look great in that. Doesn't that colour suit you? And then those that prompt people to ask if you're feeling OK. To a large extent your natural skin tone dictates the colours you should wear. As you get older – and greyer – this changes, but not in a dramatic way until you are well into old age. These days there are no set rules about what colours to put together. Virtually anything goes. If you don't feel confident with colour, take advice from someone who does – generally the person working in the shop. If you feel most comfortable in classic black, beige and white – go there. But if you like to make an impact, even if you are a size 16 or more, choose bright vibrant tops and jackets and layer them over a monochrome base.

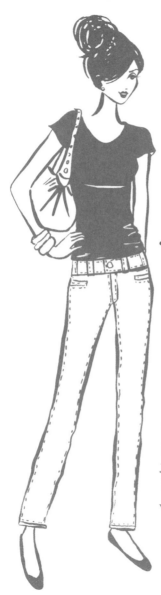

The perfect jeans...

... don't happen by luck. There's no escaping it, finding the right fit and style takes time. Be prepared to put in a few torturous hours in the changing rooms and you'll thank yourself. Because once you have the perfect pair, you'll wonder how you got along without them. Here are a few tips to take with you on the journey.

If you have a small waist but big hips and bum, there are jeans out there cut with no waistband, have a flat front and a side zip that are most flattering.

If you have shorter legs go for a boot cut. Skinny jeans will make your legs look even shorter. Slight width at the hem creates hip balance and longer-looking legs.

If you are short, be careful of Capri pants cut mid-calf because they can make you look shorter.

Unless you are slim, never wear jeans that are really tight.

★

Wear jeans with a heel for extra leg length but be mindful that really high heels pitch you forward and push out your rear end when you walk. Your bottom could look big in these..

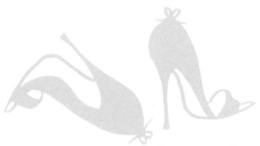

Best foot forward

When you're 20 you can get away with just about any pair of shoes – trainers, workman's boots, high rise wedges, backless stilettos – they either look sporty, funky or just plain sexy. But as you get older you find yourself paying more for a decent pair of leather shoes. First you need the comfort of something that's been properly put together, and second, like it or not, we're judged by the quality of our footwear more than just about anything else in our wardrobe. Here are seven tips for buying shoes:

1 High heels are sexy but heels that are too high tip you forward and make your bum stick out. The effect is worse if you're short.

2 As we age, the balls of our feet have less padding and we need extra cushioning. Make sure the shoes you are buying have soft inner soles or buy some of those little foam pads from the shoe shop.

3 If you are a bigger size be careful about wearing spiky stilettos. They can make you look top heavy.

4 If your ankles are thicker than you'd like them to be, don't wear ankle strap shoes or sandals with skirts.

5 Wearing towering high heels with a micro mini-skirt will make you look like a lap dancer. The rule is: the shorter the skirt the lower the heel.

6 Be careful with wedges. If you're short you can look plain silly.

7 Never sacrifice comfort for style. Chances are those pointy toe stilettos will end up gathering dust in the wardrobe.

Five 40s Fashion Faux-Pas

★ *Oversized T-shirts.*
And don't even think one with a slogan.

★ *Billowing skirts: you're not Stevie Nicks.*

★ *Spaghetti straps: too little, too late.*

★ *The wrong-shaped jeans: think muffin tops,*
short tight legs, and dare we say, pleats?

★ *Nothing but black shoes. Italian grandmother.*
Need we say more?

Age doesn't matter as much in fashion these days. But in these no-rules, wear-what-you-like, DIY personal style times, decision-making can be excruciatingly difficult. Most of us can get away with a splash of super-trendy – which equates to young – fashion. But just a splash. By the time you are in your 40s, you should be toning things down. Make sure your fashion role model is age-appropriate: you can't go too far wrong with Cate Blanchett, Audrey Hepburn or Jackie Onassis.

How young can you get away with?

Be careful of wearing too much vintage. A 1960s mini-dress can look fantastic on a fresh-faced 20-year-old, but in your 40s you might look as though you're wearing it for the second time around.

Generally avoid too short, too tight, or too much skin, and if all else fails ask a teenager. They're brutally honest and generally have finely tuned mutton-dressed-as-lamb detectors.

Emergency HELP

If it all seems too hard, you're too time-poor, you're stuck in a rut or you're struggling to know what to do with this persistently widening waist, one of the best things you can do is call in a stylist. These are professionals who can sort through your wardrobe, take you shopping and ultimately save you money. Better still, ask for one for your birthday. You'll find them in the Yellow Pages under 'Image Consultants'.

The little black dress

Synonymous with class, style, sophistication and a woman who knows her way around, the little black dress has long been the older woman's staple. To find the LBD that's best for you, first work out what shape you are. If you are an hourglass, think Sophia Loren and wow them with a fitted or crossover top with a V-neckline, a nipped-in waist and a skirt that skims out over your hips. If you have a small top and big hips you can look slim and elegant in an A-line dress, which comes in just below the bust line or above the waist and falls in a straight line out over your hips – not too flared or pencil slim. If you have broad shoulders, not much waist and slim hips, the empire line can look stunning – especially if you are tall.

A TIP: When worn too near the face, black can create dark shadows in lines and wrinkles. To avoid this draining effect, go for a scooped or V-neckline, or add some chunky, sparkly jewellery to create colour, light and movement around the face.

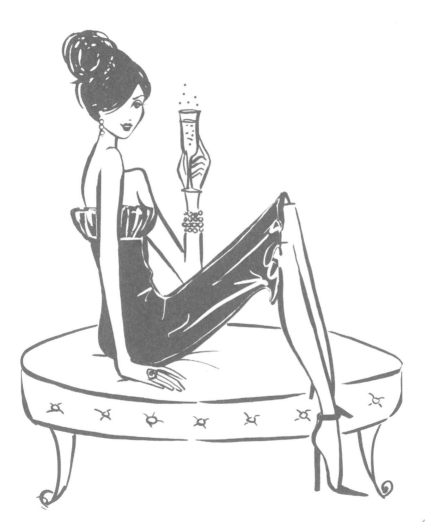

Show some leg

If you are lucky enough to have perfectly shaped pins, relish the thought that they will probably stay that way right into old age. A neatly turned ankle will see you through life. The problem lies in the detail. Our legs don't always bear close inspection. As we age, dry skin becomes more of an issue and leads to crepey calves. Then there are the dreaded crinkly knees. As our thigh muscles shrink, our once smooth knees start to develop folds and wrinkles. Next time you wonder if someone has had a facelift, check out her knees – they're a dead giveaway.

A neatly turned ankle will see you through life.

The good news is in winter you can cover them up with sheer flesh-coloured pantyhose – definitely not nude opaques, which are very old lady. Black opaques are very chic with boots, though teaming them with a black shoe that's even slightly chunky can make you look like one of the uniformed branch. Patterns and fishnets work with a knee-length skirt and heels, as do high-quality sheers. But never wear pantyhose with a shoe that has an open heel or toe.

In summer, exfoliate like mad then try one of the amazing new fake tans on well-moisturised and silky smooth legs. A golden glow can take 10 years off your legs. Technology has moved on from the days when you could smell a fake tan before you saw it. The new products are easy to use at home, or visit a salon for a professional application. Look for easy-to-apply mousses, spray-ons (these need practice) and the useful moisturiser/tan combos that add colour subtly and gradually.

A TIP: As with everything else in cosmetic medicine, treatment for varicose veins has been getting less invasive in recent years. Now, sclerotherapy — once only used for dealing with smaller spider veins and broken capillaries — has been developed to be effective on the biggies. For these procedures it is best to go to a phlebologist — a doctor who specialises in veins.

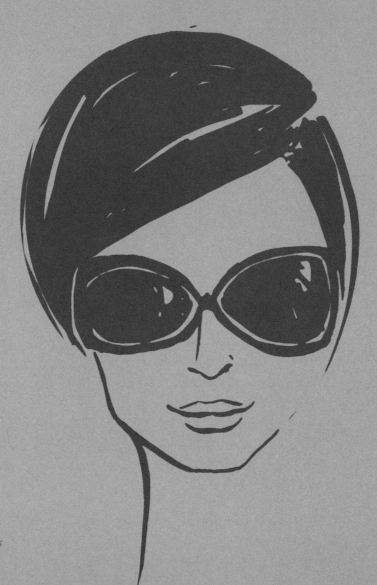

When you find yourself ordering what you hope is
the goat's cheese but it could be the grilled quail, it's
time to explore the world of specs. Visit an optometrist
to find out what your prescription is, and then treat
yourself to some gorgeous designer frames. Be brave,
and maybe get a pair for day and one for evening. If
you're one of the lucky ones who only needs a tiny bit
of magnification, you can start with some of the funky-
framed magnifying specs they sell over the counter in
pharmacies. There are some very stylish frames around
and they're cheap enough that you can buy plenty of
pairs to leave around the house, car and office so that
you're never caught out.

Eye spy – or I don't

Cheap sunglasses from high-street fashion stores are
a brilliant way to add an up-to-the-minute angle to an
outfit. You can even take them to your optometrist to
have lenses in your prescription added.

Comfy cups

Our breasts change size and shape throughout life and we should be regularly checking that we are wearing the right size and fit. Of course, many of us soldier on with the bra that we've always bought. So if you are constantly readjusting your underwear all day you're probably wearing the wrong size. A bra should feel so comfortable that you forget it's there.

For a great fit, ensure the back strap fits snugly and sits firmly – otherwise it's not doing its job of supporting the breasts. It shouldn't ride up or be so slack that your breasts fall out of the front.

TRY THIS: When you first buy a bra, fasten it on the loosest hook, so as it stretches with wear you can tighten the hooks as you go. This gives you a bit more life out of the bra.

If the shoulder straps dig in, it could be because your back strap is too loose, leaving your breasts inadequately supported, which leads you to overtighten the shoulder straps to compensate.

The cup should encompass the entire breast – there shouldn't be anything squishing over the top or around the sides. It's very common to have one breast larger than the other, if this is your situation, choose the cup size that fits the larger breast.

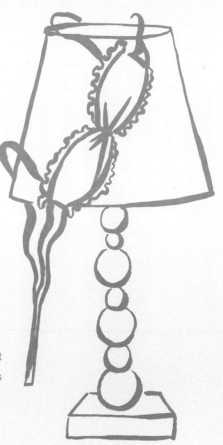

The best thing about handbags is that they are fashion items we can all enjoy no matter what shape and size we are and at any age. We can express our personality and mood through them. They tell the world who we are. Are you a tan leather and fringe sort of person, a neat black clasp and over the arm type lady or a slouchy, unstructured, hang it off the shoulder kind of girl?

Best bags

Thankfully the matching shoes and bag days have long gone. But now it's all about the fearfully expensive signature bag. And when every A-lister is hauling around a Hermès Birkin or the very latest Louis Vuitton Mahina bag, it's tempting to trade in the car and jump on the bandwagon. But stop right there and ask yourself just one question: where will you take it? If you work in the fashion or advertising industries you can get away with telling yourself it's a career investment. But if you toil undetected in accounts or childcare or just about anywhere else and spend your spare time watching junior soccer or taking the dog for a walk, and have a mortgage, stick to a mid price range bag.

Don't go for cheap unless it's a wild and colourful statement and you have the personality to carry it off. If you are on a budget, buy from the discount outlets of the better manufacturers. If you must have a designer logo, try eBay and the second-hand designer or vintage clothes shops.

Four bags you must have:

1   A timeless classically shaped bag with good lines in the best leather.

2   The stylish weekend hold-all that can take you shopping, to the beach and even double as an overnighter. It can take the pressure off your more expensive 'classic' bag.

3   A slim, elegant evening envelope or clutch bag – either black or something sparkly – that can go with everything.

4   Something fun or exotic that expresses your wilder side.

These days jewellery is more fun than it used to be.

There's nothing more dating than jewellery that's a decade out of step or piled on. Since bling became a big part of American street culture, heavy gold jewellery has become most passé in ladylike places. It's all about platinum and diamonds or silver and cubic zirconias – depending on your budget. If you can't afford Tiffany there are some great fakes around that come with a lifetime guarantee. These days jewellery is more fun than it used to be. Pile on the beads if you want to let loose. But buy them from designer gift and craft shops – that way you won't see them on everyone else.

Gilt trip

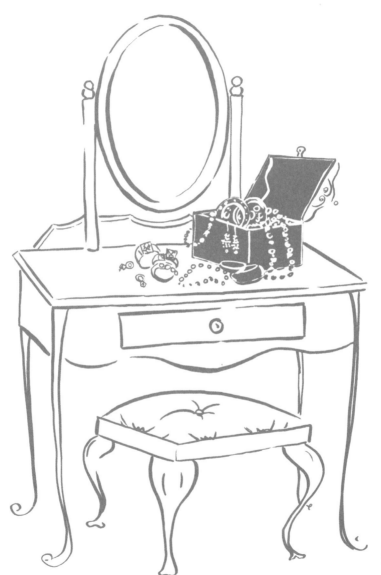

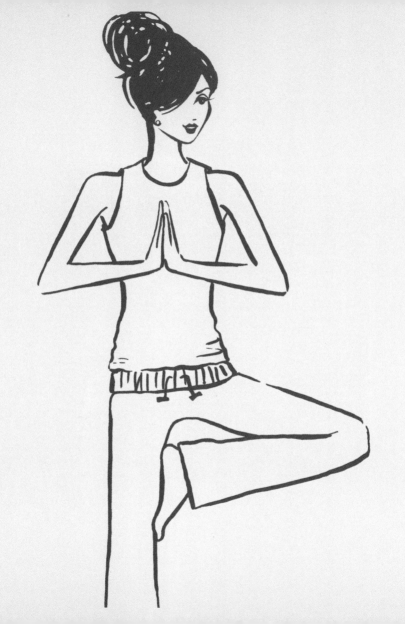

Body

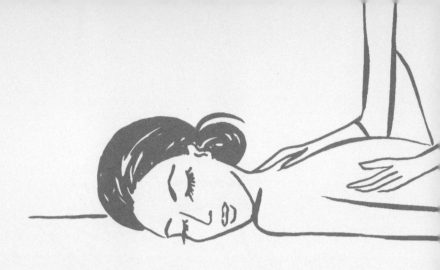

*a*t 40 you have a mission: to make sure that you slim down to racing weight so you can emerge from menopause looking svelte and superb. You might have found weight has crept on slowly over the years. Maybe you never lost that extra baby weight; or a cosy relationship has meant snug nights at home eating comfort food together; or perhaps you've been deskbound for 20 years and hardly had time to walk to the car, let alone visit a gym.

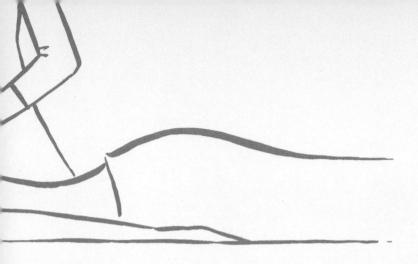

Tough but true

There is no kind way to say this, so here goes. If you are overweight in your 40s you'd better start getting serious about shaping up and slimming down – and quickly. In the run-up to menopause most women find maintaining weight becomes more difficult, and losing the extra padding becomes almost impossible. Do yourself a favour, and start menopause as slim as you can be. This way you stand a better chance of staying that way.

Check out your BMI

Your Body Mass Index is the measurement that gives a true reading of how fat you are and therefore how healthy you are. Figure it out by dividing your weight in kilograms by your height in metres squared. If you aren't a maths whiz, you'll find that quite a few of the bigger pharmacies or your GP will measure it for you, or use one of the many online BMI calculators.

Carrying excess weight around your middle is more harmful than having hip and thigh fat. Abdominal fat increases the risk of heart disease.

Underweight = less than 18.5

Normal weight = 18.5–24.9

Overweight = 25–29.9

Obese = 30 or greater

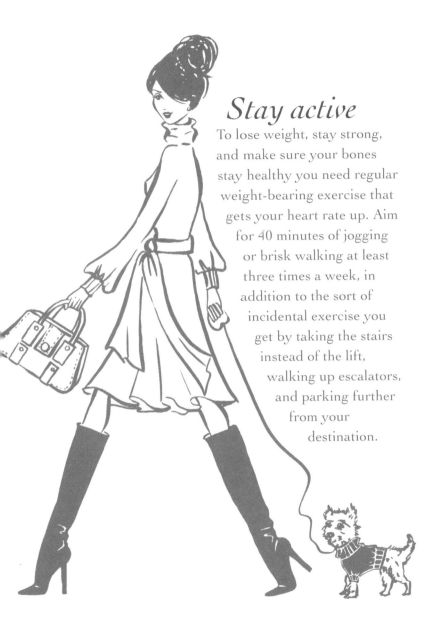

Stay active

To lose weight, stay strong, and make sure your bones stay healthy you need regular weight-bearing exercise that gets your heart rate up. Aim for 40 minutes of jogging or brisk walking at least three times a week, in addition to the sort of incidental exercise you get by taking the stairs instead of the lift, walking up escalators, and parking further from your destination.

NOTE IT: Keep a food diary – a completely honest record of what you consume. The results may surprise you. After a week, review your daily eating habits and look at how you can cut back a little further.

REDUCE IT: Slash about 400 kilojoules from your daily diet and you should be able to start losing weight. Just skip the biscuits at morning tea, or swap that glass of wine for a sparkling mineral water.

SHOP SMART: It can be hard with a family, but try to avoid buying nutritionally empty foods. If you don't buy biscuits and chips you can't eat them. Try not to shop for groceries on an empty stomach.

Dieting may be difficult but it's not rocket science. The extra kilos came on gradually, and so will the weight loss. Just make some small changes that really add up.

SLEEP IT OFF: Lack of sleep increases the levels of a hunger hormone and decreases levels of a hormone that makes you feel full. So try to get a good night's sleep every night.

MOVE IT: Exercise is the real key to weight loss. Start small and work up from there, but most importantly, make moving a part of your life.

COMMIT TO IT: Don't rush at weight loss like a bull in a china shop. The people who successfully lose weight take a steady approach and lose it over a few months or even years. What you are aiming for is to reprogram your life habits.

So what's stopping you?

It is truly difficult to lose weight without increasing your exercise. Not only does exercise burn calories, but it also increases your metabolism so you'll burn more calories even when you're resting. And its mood-improving capabilities are an added bonus. Talk to anybody who runs or cycles regularly and they'll tell you how the endorphins kick in and it becomes addictive.

Getting to grips with exercise

Any exercise is better than none at all. The first step is always the hardest and you'll be amazed how much easier it gets over time. A ten-minute walk to the shops and back is a great start and remember, the more exercise you do the better your chance of losing weight.

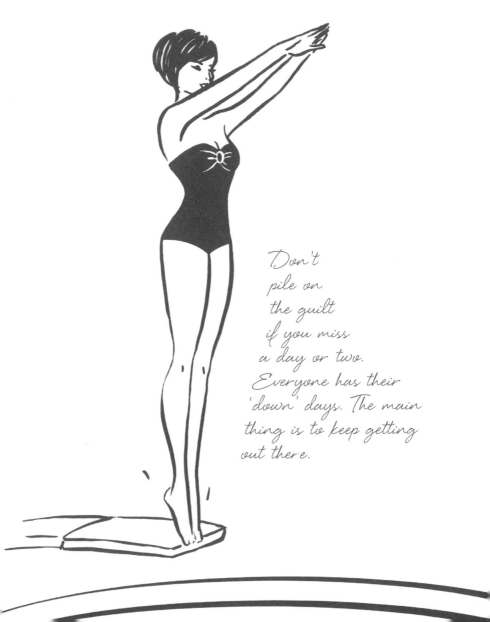

Don't
pile on
the guilt
if you miss
a day or two.
Everyone has their
'down' days. The main
thing is to keep getting
out there.

Mix it up

The best exercise is one you enjoy. Take an iPod with you or go with a friend. Walk by the river, through the park – even take a brisk walk through your local shopping mall. Look for ways to build activity into your life. Find a sport or activity the whole family can enjoy. It could bring you closer together. Think cycling, walking, swimming, golf, tennis, soccer, volleyball, and good old backyard cricket. It's all exercise. Park further away from the shopping centre or work; take the stairs, not the lift.

Saved by stretching

You're flexible in every other area of life – juggling work, family and friends – so why forget your body? As you age, muscles and joints tend to become tighter and less able to move. It's much easier to maintain flexibility while you still have it, so start stretching now. Exercises that combine stretching with weight bearing – like yoga or Pilates – are ideal, but don't forget you need cardio too for weight loss and heart health.

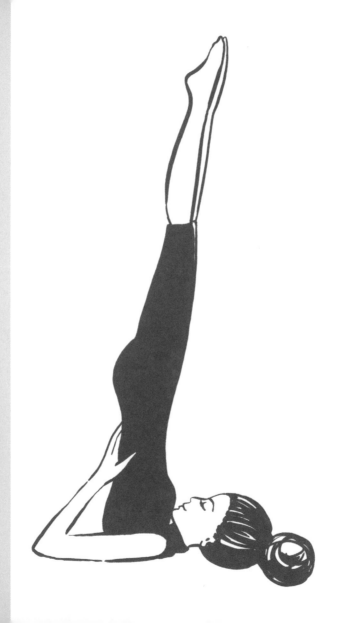

83

Lift your game

The first thing you need to know is that weight training doesn't equal bodybuilding. If you start lifting weights you won't automatically turn into a rippling hulk. Weightlifting, done properly and regularly, increases the lean muscle mass, which speeds metabolism and helps you burn fat. Working out with weights also helps sculpt a gorgeous shape, which you will see emerge as the cardio burns off the fat.

TOP TIPS FOR GETTING MOVING

1 Schedule exercise in your diary. It is not an indulgence, it's a necessity. Treat it as you would another important appointment.

2 If exercise eats into your precious time with family and friends, involve them too. Go for a walk after dinner with your partner, play with the kids in the park or catch up with a girlfriend for a bike ride.

3 Too tired? Tell yourself you only have to exercise for 10 minutes. You'll probably find after 10 minutes you'll feel like continuing.

4 Integrate weight and stretching into your life: bicep curls with heavy shopping bags, a few lunges while waiting for the shower to heat up – it's amazing how creative you'll be when you get started.

Fashions in diets come and go . . .

. . . high-protein, low-carb, low GI, macrobiotic, Pritikin, Atkins, South Beach, the Zone – they have all had their time in the spotlight. High-protein meals can crank up your metabolism for a brief period, but they aren't sustainable and they aren't good for your general health.

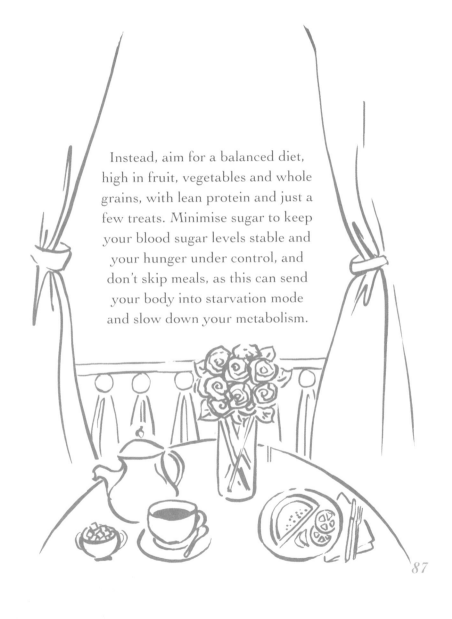

Instead, aim for a balanced diet, high in fruit, vegetables and whole grains, with lean protein and just a few treats. Minimise sugar to keep your blood sugar levels stable and your hunger under control, and don't skip meals, as this can send your body into starvation mode and slow down your metabolism.

Reward yourself

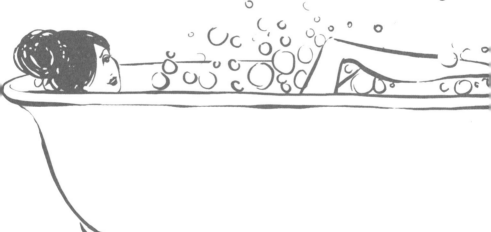

Party tricks

Socialising when you are eating healthily doesn't have to be hard. Stick to veggies dipped in low-fat dips like hummus, or better still, eat before a party so you aren't as tempted by the canapés. You'll lose weight faster if you don't drink, but if you do, alternate mineral water and alcoholic drinks. If you drink mixed drinks, avoid sugary soft fizzies as mixers.

If you've managed to survive the week without raiding the fridge in the middle of the night or sneaking biscuits at work, find a way to reward yourself that doesn't involve food. The best substitutes involve something physically pleasant – like a massage, a facial, a hot bath, listening to music, or sex, if there is someone close at hand.

TOP TIPS FOR KEEPING TRIM

Go plain: *skip butter, sauces and mayonnaise.
You don't need them.*

Choose fish over meat: *an average steak
is about 2000kj. Grilled fish is about 1000kj.*

Eat protein: *it keeps you feeling fuller longer.*

Learn to love salads:
they are a slimmer's best friend.

Say no to cake:
just a slice could be as much as 1000kj.

Be careful *of foods labelled 'lite'
and '...% fat free': lite can mean how
a product looks or feels, and 96% fat free = 4% fat.
Whole milk has 4% fat and isn't considered a diet food.*

Balancing act

Losing weight doesn't have to mean giving up all the things you love. It's just a question of balance. Here are some ways to compensate for indulging in the finer things.

A glass of wine	=	15 minute jog
A dark chocolate truffle	=	30 minutes walking the dog
A Magnum ice-cream	=	1.5 hours pushing a child in a stroller
A croissant	=	50 minutes on an exercise bike

Why not swap some high-kilojoule foods and beverages for low? You probably won't even notice the difference.

Caffè latte with whole milk	545kj
Caffè latte with skim milk (less than 1 percent fat)	335kj
Filter coffee with whole milk	85kj
Long black	35kj
Instant coffee with low fat milk (2 per cent fat)	90kj
Tea with whole milk	90kj
Tea with skim milk	55kj

If you are a regular drinker, a straightforward way to lose weight is to stop or reduce your drinking. For many of us, having a couple of glasses of wine in the evening is a pleasant way to end a stressful work day. The trouble is that a glass of wine at home is rarely the 100ml standard drink, it's usually 1.5 to 2.5 standard drinks. This means that 'a couple' ends up being half a bottle. Half a bottle of wine is about 1570 kilojoules. Add a few crackers and cheese and you've wrecked your diet in one sitting.

Tough but true: Is alcohol making you fat?

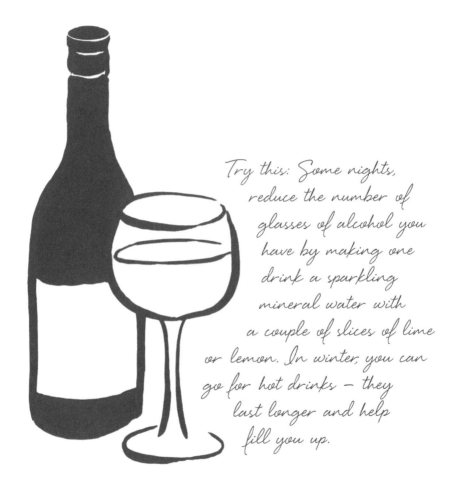

Try this: Some nights, reduce the number of glasses of alcohol you have by making one drink a sparkling mineral water with a couple of slices of lime or lemon. In winter, you can go for hot drinks — they last longer and help fill you up.

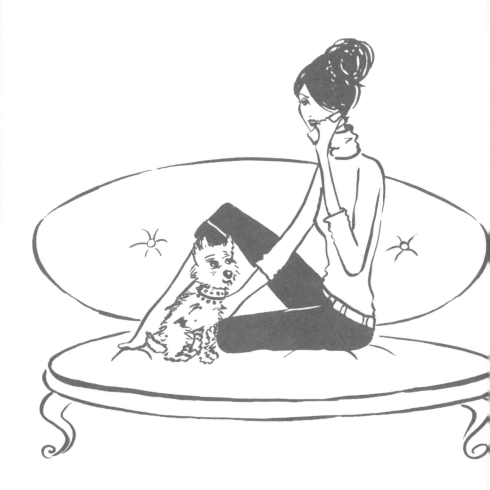

Calling for back-up

If you're struggling, call in the cavalry. Weight Watchers, Jenny Craig and a host of other organisations can help you get back on the right track. Some groups run support online – great for those who don't want to front up to meetings. Nutritionists are a valuable source of expert information. Some people use hypnotherapy to help them stay motivated. Your GP can prescribe medications. Just don't be afraid to ask.

Some people use hypnotherapy to help them stay motivated.

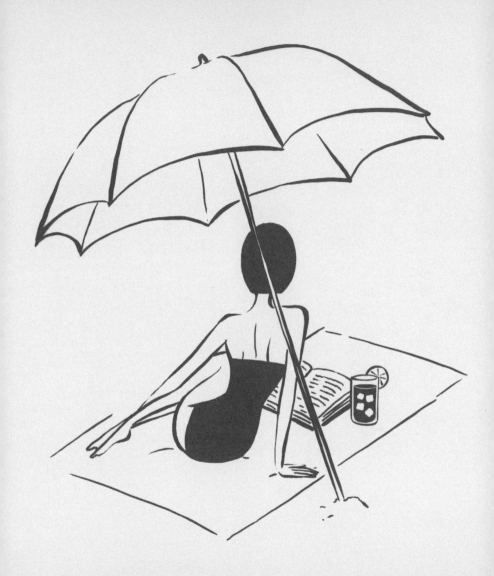

Health

*B*y the time you get to your 40s there are days when you dare to feel that you're finally getting the hang of life. You've had enough hard knocks to know that you're actually quite resilient – and proud of it. You're doing OK at work. Partnered or single, you've a fair idea of what you want out of a relationship. You've never felt more confident or strong. Then over the horizon looms menopause.

Things seriously start changing from that point, so use your 40s to get yourself in great shape to minimise the impact of ageing and menopause.

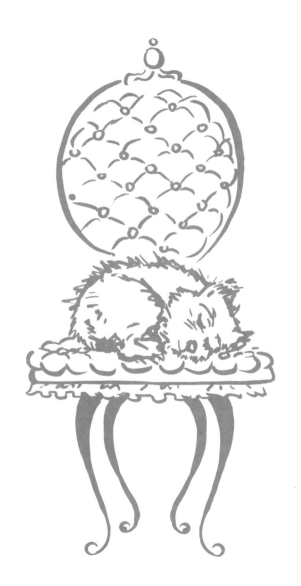

Change is a-comin'

There are subtle changes to your body for up to 10 years before menopause and this transitional time is called perimenopause. The average age of menopause is about 51, with most women experiencing it somewhere between 45 and 55. And here's a thought: perimenopause can begin as early as your mid to late 30s.

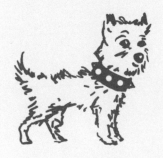

Oestrogen and progesterone levels rise and fall unevenly and you begin having cycles in which you don't ovulate. With so many hormones crashing about and then disappearing altogether for a while, it's not surprising that emotionally things can be rocky: you might feel irritable; have a decreased sex drive; or have problems sleeping. Sounds fabulous, doesn't it?

How you live life in perimenopause can make a big difference not only to how you cope with the symptoms of menopause but how healthy you are afterwards. If there was ever a time in life to eat a healthy diet and take up some exercise it's now. Any exercise can make a difference – a brisk walk, an hour's stretching. Some people find yoga very beneficial. Your GP can be a great ally.

When the first hot flushes hit . . .

. . . the urge is strong to find something to stop them. But taking medication – whether a pill or a so-called natural supplement – is now one of the most controversial topics in women's health. There's no easy answer and even with all of the medical advice and Googling in the world, in the end you have to make your own decision. Who said menopause was easy?

Once Hormone Replacement Therapy (HRT) was regarded as a youth pill – something that would miraculously help us stay younger longer – but there is no real evidence to support this. HRT is certainly effective for slowing osteoporosis and if this is a problem you need to discuss the pros and cons with your doctor. The problem is that many long and intensive studies around the world have continued to link HRT with breast cancer. The studies have also shown a stronger link between HRT and stroke in older women. As you can imagine, there is probably no other topic as hotly debated at medical conferences around the world.

There are plenty of non-pharmaceutical methods of relieving the symptoms of menopause. Some of the oldest and most popular are:

Going herbal?

Black Cohosh: This is probably the most useful of the herbal products. It's long been used by native Americans for menstrual cramps and menopausal symptoms and is the most researched of all herbs used for the management of menopause. Trials have shown it to be effective in helping reduce hot flushes and reducing vaginal dryness. Taking too much can lead to toxicity, and a few cases of liver damage have been reported in Australia. Black Cohosh has also been used in trials as a way of treating hot flushes for breast cancer survivors.

Wild Yam Cream:

This is not a progesterone and cannot be converted to progesterone in the body. It contains diosgenin that can be converted in a laboratory to the sort of progesterone and oestrogen found in the pill and HRT but not the same progesterone found naturally in the body.

Evening Primrose Oil:

This is widely used for hot flushes and often prescribed by health professionals, but studies have shown it to be no better than a placebo at relieving hot flushes.

A TIP: Experimenting with over-the-counter preparations may be more costly than seeing a trained herbalist or naturopath. Some herbal products may contain herbs that should not be used in conjunction with pharmaceutical hormone therapies but they do not carry any warning. The other problem with the 'natural' therapies is that they are less regulated than pharmaceutically based medications, so there is less evidence available to show if and how well they work.

Four health checks to have in your 40s

1 **BREAST CHECKS:** the Cancer Council recommends you to be breast aware and see your GP if you notice anything unusual. Once you are 40 you can attend the Breast Screen Australia program but it isn't free until you hit 50.

2 **PAP SMEARS:** if you have ever been sexually active you must have one every two years.

3 **CHOLESTEROL AND TRIGLYCERIDES BLOOD TEST:** have one every five years in your 40s because you are at greater risk of hardening of the arteries and heart attacks (more frequently if there is a family history). Have your blood pressure taken every 18 months or more often if you have a family history of high blood pressure.

4 **FASTING BLOOD SUGAR LEVEL:** if you are overweight or have a family history of diabetes, have a test every three years.

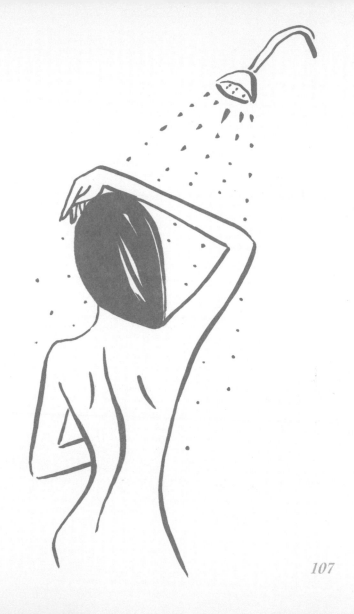

Great bones

As oestrogen levels fall, so does protection against bone loss, so make sure you are getting enough calcium. The recommended daily dietary intake of calcium for women is 1000–1300 milligrams. Most of us are unlikely to achieve this through our normal diet alone, so supplements can be useful. They can slow bone loss, although they do not completely stop it. Too much caffeine can accelerate bone loss, so try to limit your intake. Find out more about calcium from your GP. If there are symptoms of osteoporosis, you may be sent for a bone density scan.

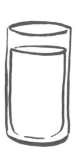

Don't wait until you are in your 50s or 60s to start thinking about cholesterol. The earlier you start working to prevent it the better. High cholesterol increases your risk of stroke and heart disease.

Once you hit 45 you should have a cholesterol and triglycerides blood test every five years. Cut down on saturated fats such as fatty meat and dairy products like butter, cheese and cream. Go for low-fat dairy products, spreads that have been designed to counteract high cholesterol, olive oil, avocados, oats, soy products, seeds and nuts.

Cut your cholesterol

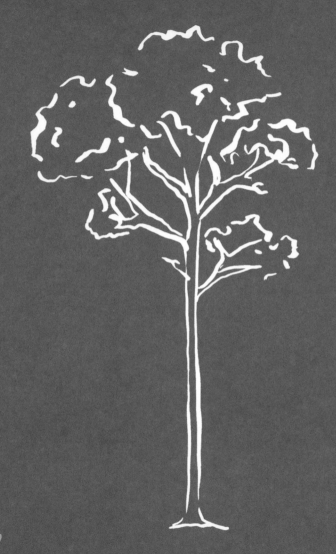

By 2010, lung cancer will overtake breast cancer as the biggest killer of Australian women. Although treatment for lung cancer is slowly improving, it kills more of its victims than any other cancer. And far from keeping you

Tough but true: lung cancer

slim, scientists have discovered that smoking probably interferes with the body's metabolism and triggers it to store more fat. The only thing you can do to minimise the risk of lung cancer is stop smoking now. Start by seeing your doctor, who can help devise a program and suggest some courses of action, including behavioural therapy, medication, self-help programs, hypnosis and acupuncture.

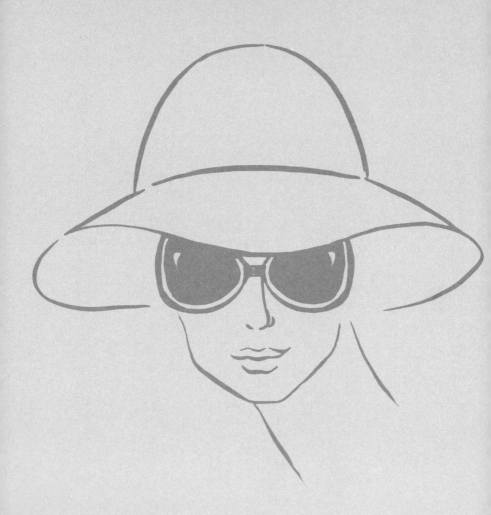

10 things you can do to reduce your risk of cancer

1. Aim for a BMI of 21 to 23 and avoid gaining weight.

2. Take about 40 minutes of moderate exercise daily – like brisk walking.

3. Avoid junk food and sugary drinks.

4. Eat no more than 500 grams of red meat a week and avoid processed meats altogether.

5. Limit daily alcohol intake to one standard drink.

6. Eat five portions of non-starchy vegetables and two portions of fruit daily.

7. Avoid salt-preserved food. Limit salt intake to 6 grams daily.

8. Don't smoke.

9. Breastfeed your babies for 6 months.

10. Stay out of the sun.

This is currently the most common cancer for Australian women, but the good news is that thanks to earlier diagnoses and new treatment regimes, survival rates have improved by more than 25 percent in the last decade.

Breast cancer

Your risk of developing breast cancer increases with risk factors such as obesity, not having children or having them later in life, long-term use of HRT, intake of alcohol, eating a diet high in red meat and fat. Numerous research studies have shown that women who undertake moderate exercise and watch their diet can reduce their risk.

Try this: Limit meat dishes to two or three times a week and buy a couple of good veggie cookbooks.

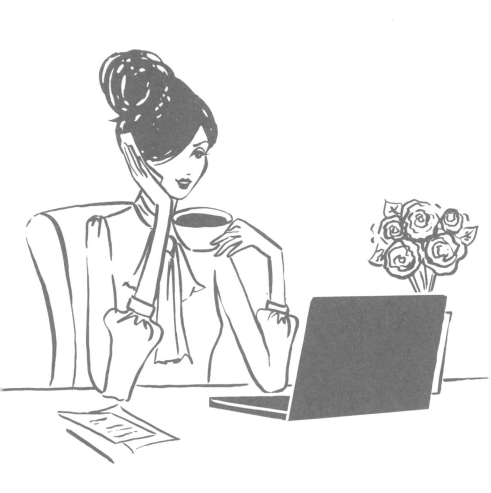

Computer back

One of the best things you can do for yourself when you hit your 40s is to sort out any posture problems. If you are among the many thousands who spend their work days bent over a computer for hours on end you'll need to take action to avoid ending up with a rounded back and shoulders – always a tell-tale sign of old ladydom. Get yourself checked out by a good musculo-skeletal or remedial therapist or physio. They can check your posture and straighten you out with exercises and manipulation.

TRY THIS: When sitting for long periods, stand up and roll your neck and shoulders at least once an hour to help the body maintain circulation and to lubricate the muscles and joints.

Twisting the body can relieve backaches, headaches and stiffness and can be done in a sitting or standing position. As the trunk turns, the kidneys and abdominal organs are activated and exercised. The spine becomes flexible and the hips move more easily. Breathe with the movement.

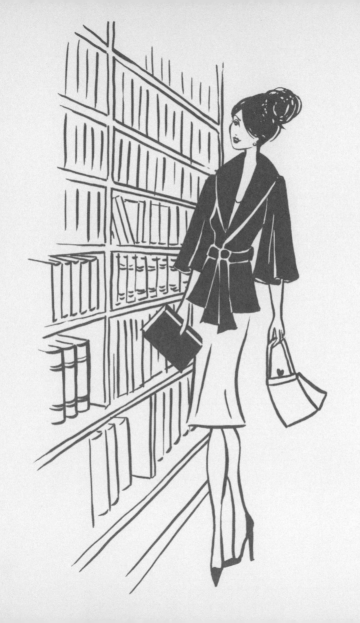

Living

*I*f there was such a thing as the award for the most stressful decade, the 40s would win it hands down. By now you are so good at managing kids, partner and career that everyone is piling you up with more things to do. At work you're known as Mrs Responsible and you always follow through – so you get the extra or tricky jobs. Your partner needs your support because he is at a stage where he has his own life/career decisions to make. The kids are heading for the dreaded early teens. And to top it off, your parents are newly retired and making more demands on your time – for better or worse. Then there are those 40s who've just gone through a major life crisis and are picking themselves up after divorce or are trying to make a relationship work. Whatever your situation, the 40s is the time for some urgent stocktaking and some intensive 'me' therapy. Read on . . .

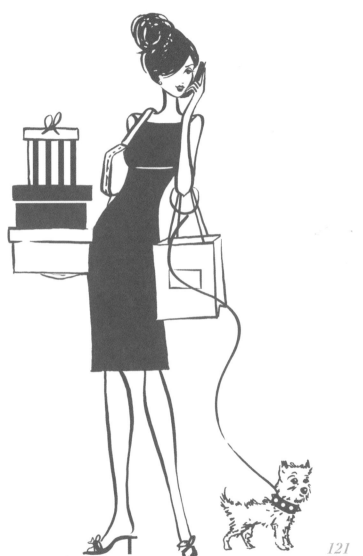

How much time do you spend thinking about the things you are going to do … one day? Do you initiate things in your life or do you just react? Do the weekends pass in a blur while you rush around just trying to get on top of things so you can hurtle to work again on Monday? Do you never have anything to wear because you haven't had time to go through your wardrobe? Do you feel that life is slipping by quicker than you'd like?

Planning your life

It could be time for some personal planning. Finding out who you are and what you want to achieve is a way of reaching your full potential.

ASK YOURSELF

How do you spend your time?

★

*What do you feel about the things
in your life that you do?*

★

How important are they?

★

*Are there things you hate doing
and activities you love?*

★

*What would you choose to do if you had
no obligations to anyone?*

★

Prioritise

Your answers can tell you a lot about yourself and what is important to you. Once you've worked out what they are, try to build these aspirations into your life. Make a list of the things you do in order of what is most important to you. Set some goals and plan step by step how you can achieve them in set time frames. What positive actions do you need? What are you prepared to sacrifice? What are the likely risks?

Indulge

Do yourself a favour – be selfish. People who are selfish live longer. So when life seems tough and the going is harder than ever, just stop for a minute and do something nice for yourself. Most importantly, don't feel guilty about it.

Spend a day or half a day doing what you want to do – not what the family wants or work dictates.

Stay in bed an extra hour or watch a movie in bed.

Drop into your local coffee shop and watch
the passing parade.

Get out the old photos and take a trip down memory lane.

Book a massage, or a full-day or half-day of beauty treatment.

Buy a couple of magazines and lie in the garden
(but don't get up to mow it).

Browse through your favourite shop or market.

Time for a boost

It's the pitter-patter of tiny defeats: every now and then in life something happens to make us lose confidence. Someone at the office makes a snide remark; uncomfortably, your 'other half' seems distracted; the man at the dry cleaners is downright rude. You feel used and abused. These are the times for some psychological first aid:

Spend 15 minutes thinking about the good things that have happened in life – what people said about you at your 30th or 40th birthday or when you left your last job.

★

Step into your friends' shoes and try to see why they like you and why they keep in touch with you.

★

Think about the clever things you did as a child and how your mum was so proud of that painting, that poem or that song you sang.

★

Make a mental list of all your good qualities.

★

Stop comparing yourself to others. It's irrational and can be habit-forming.

Taking back time

Juggling a career with partner, kids and social life? Welcome to the world of the 40-something. Although everyone seems to be working longer and harder than ever, the poor Ms 40 cops more than her fair share and is punching way above her weight – which is precisely why more of us are starting to ask ourselves how on earth we got here. Work–life balance has become the buzz phrase but every now and then there is an uncomfortable feeling that it's probably just empty rhetoric thought up by an underworked HR department.

Or consider DOWNSIZING – moving to a less expensive house in a smaller town where there is less pressure and more time to smell the flowers.

OPTIONS

BE BRAVE and say 'No'. Work the hours you're paid to do and don't be pressured into staying longer.

WORK PART-TIME and forgo the higher salary for more time with your family.

JOB SHARE where you can.

CHANGE YOUR CAREER for something with less responsibility.

IF YOUR CAREER IS A PRIORITY, get help at home.

DITCH THE 'TO DO' LIST – because therein lies the path to madness. Unless you can finish it in a day, leave it till tomorrow.

LOOK AFTER YOUR HEALTH and remind yourself that this is the most important thing in your life.

REWARD YOURSELF for working hard. Otherwise what's the point?

Learning to delegate

As women, we're not naturals at delegating – while often men are. Put it down to genes, hormones, conditioning or just our innate ability to multi-task, but for the majority of us it's easy to go into overdrive and whirl around making other people's lives a misery while we 'get things done'. As nurturers we tend to slip into responsibility mode all too easily. It's amazing that when we're rushed off our feet to the point of exhaustion we still can't let someone else take some of the burden. If only we could, our lives might be so much happier, less stressed – and possibly longer. Here are a few tips for lightening the load:

LET GO OF THE NEED TO BE IN CONTROL.
Once you can do this you'll be amazed at how
good you feel and how liberated.

ADMIT THAT YOU'RE NOT INDISPENSABLE.
None of us is, so get over it.

ACCEPT THAT SOMEONE ELSE CAN DO THE JOB
and think of it as an opportunity rather than a threat.

LETTING OTHER PEOPLE HELP CAN MAKE THEM FEEL
GOOD, which can make you feel good.

OUTSOURCE THE JOBS YOU HATE.
Get a cleaner once a fortnight, an ironing person,
a gardener once a month, and drive through the
car wash or pay the kid up the road to do it.

Five tips for preserving emotional energy

We can all easily get overloaded with other people's problems. It's the way we're made. How often have you found yourself swamped and emotionally drained because you felt duty-bound to rescue somebody or buoy them up when they had an unpleasant issue to handle. The chances are they breezed off feeling much better while you were left strung out or downright depressed. It's good to support friends and family – but within reason. If you don't take control you can easily end up feeling depressed and victimised.

1 **You are not responsible for the happiness of others.** *Keep reminding yourself, this is important.*

2 **For some people complaining is just a habit.** *Recognise this and don't take them too seriously.*

3 **Don't feel obliged to say 'yes'.** *In fact practise saying 'no' to people who constantly overload you with responsibility.*

4 **Don't do favours that are beyond the call.** *If it's something that you wouldn't reasonably ask of someone else, why do it?*

5 **Practise saying 'no' nicely.** *Once you've mastered this you will feel upbeat and in control.*

Finding Mr or Ms Right in your 40s

There are many women who love being single because they have the freedom to do what they want, as well as total financial independence, and all the time in the world to devote to a career or other pursuits. But it's no fun being on your own if you don't want to be.

By the time you get to 40 you probably have a fair idea of who you are. If you've been through a divorce or separation you'll also be amazingly resilient. But even the most intelligent, funny, commonsensical and fabulous-looking women seem to go coy at the prospect of finding Mr or Ms Right. And the trouble is, you won't find him or her by sitting at home watching *Law and Order* in your PJs with a glass of wine in your hand.

In every other aspect of your life, once you've decided you want something you make plans to get it; so why not relationships? Apply a few business principles to finding a partner. Work out what you've got to offer the market, how best to package it up, identify who you are interested in merging with, and then make your approach.

Make a list
of the qualities you want from a partner and
prioritise.

Remember nobody's perfect,
so be prepared to accept a percentage of your
wish list.

Go places
where people of both sexes hang out. If you want a
millionaire, join the sailing group at your local yacht
club; if you want a spunk, join the gym.

Hunt in a pack:
it's easier to go places with a group of friends.

But most importantly:

Dont get desperate: it's unattractive in either sex.

Get a life of your own: if you're happy and fulfilled you'll find men falling out of the trees.

Don't lie about your children: if he doesn't want kids around, you could be setting yourself up for a huge heartache.

And never forget that being single is far better than being in an unhappy relationship.

Broaden your horizons

Work, home, partner, kids, family, friends, work, home, partner . . . does it ever feel like you are on a not-so-merry-go-round? As much as you love all these aspects of your life, do you sometimes feel as if it's always just the same old same old? Injecting inspiration into your routine doesn't have to be that hard, it just takes little steps, and occasionally trying to think outside the box.

To snap yourself out of the day-to-day doldrums, why not try:

Walking or driving home via a different route on a day when time is not too pressing?

Trying a different supermarket, or set of shops.

Changing your radio station. Even if you hate it and change back after a few hours, you've opened your mind to an alternative.

Taking your family somewhere they've never been: a new park, museum or beach.

The 40s is the time for the mid-life career change. This is the decade when the kids gain more independence and parents start re-assessing their own lives.

Take stock and plan to change

A generation ago, people were applauded and awarded if they stayed with the same employer for their whole working lives. Nowadays, the notion of a job for life has been turned on its head. You are more likely to be praised for changing careers because you can bring fresh ideas and ways of doing things to the workplace.

If you haven't been happy in your career up until now, it may be time for a re-think.

Perhaps your job feels superficial and you want to do something that will make the world a better place. ASK YOURSELF: who do I want to help? How can I put my skills and experience to good use? Do I have a passion to help children, animals, the elderly, the less advantaged or the sick?

★

It may be time to go back to college or university to train for a completely different career. ASK YOURSELF: what have I always wanted to do? Can I retrain for this career? What steps do I need to take?

★

You're fed up with being a wage slave: you want to call the shots and work for yourself or run your own business. ASK YOURSELF: what skills do I have that are marketable? What venture capital do I need to start my business? Who would give me support?

Forge Ahead

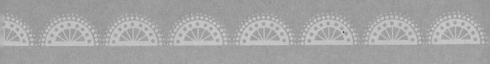

Don't think that you're over the hill at 40 – you're just reaching the summit. It's important to realise that at your age, you're probably not even halfway through your allotted lifespan. There's plenty of time in front of you for new careers, relationships and adventures. No-one can be the perfect mum, wife and employee – so work out what's best for you, and be sure to include time for yourself in the equation. One day, you'll look back and thank yourself for it.

An Ebury Press book
Published by Random House Australia Pty Ltd
Level 3, 100 Pacific Highway, North Sydney, NSW 2060
www.randomhouse.com.au

First published by Ebury Press in 2008

Addresses for companies within the Random House Group can be found at
www.randomhouse.com.au/offices.

National Library of Australia
Cataloguing-in-Publication Entry

Robson, Pamela.
Grown-up & gorgeous in your 40s.

ISBN 978 1 74166 801 8 (pbk.)

Beauty, Personal.
Women – Health and hygiene.
Middle-aged women – Health and hygiene.

646.7042

Cover and internal illustrations by Megan Hess
Cover design by Christabella Designs
Internal design by Anna Warren, Warren Ventures Pty Ltd
Additional design by Liz Seymour, Seymour Designs
Printed and bound by Tien Wah Press (PTE), Singapore

Random House Australia uses papers that are natural, renewable and recyclable products and made
from wood grown in sustainable forests. The logging and manufacturing processes are expected to
conform to the environmental regulations of the country of origin.

10 9 8 7 6 5 4 3 2